The book of Glucose Revolution

:

Blood Glucose Balance's Metabolic Potential

By

Vernon J. Shuman

TABLE OF CONTENTS

Introduction

Without seeing a doctor beforehand, do not alter your diet if you are on any medication, as this will require medication adjustment to prevent excessively low blood sugar levels (hypoglycemia). A hazardous side effect of taking too many medications is hypoglycemia.

Because this method for reversing diabetes is so successful, it is even more crucial to speak with a doctor who is informed with the drug reduction required as a result of aggressive dietary changes. Do not undervalue the effectiveness of this programme because, in the absence of drug decreases, taking too much medication could result in a dangerous hypoglycemia reaction.Many physicians, not realizing how effective this diet style is, may be hesitant

Without seeing a doctor beforehand, do not alter your diet if you are on any medication, as this will require medication adjustment to prevent excessively low blood sugar levels (hypoglycemia). A hazardous side effect of taking too many medications is hypoglycemia.

Because this method for reversing diabetes is so successful, it is even more crucial to speak with a doctor who is informed with the drug reduction required as a result of aggressive dietary changes. Do not undervalue the effectiveness of this programme because, in the absence of drug decreases, taking too much medication could result in a dangerous hypoglycemia reaction.

Chapter 1 : what is the glucose revolution ?

1. The glucose revolution's concept

The phrase "glucose revolution" is frequently used to describe the social and economic changes that took place in the French and English West Indies in the middle of the seventeenth century. Jessie Inchauspe, a researcher and author, claims that up to 90% of us have an excess of glucose in our bodies. She created her 10 hacks, which she claims are based on the most recent scientific research. They offer straightforward lifestyle tips that can help reverse the symptoms of high blood sugar levels without requiring you to go on a "diet" or give up your favorite foods.

2. Sugar oxidation

Glucose oxidation refers to the breakdown of glucose when oxygen is present. Anaerobic oxidation is the phrase used when there is no oxygen present, whereas aerobic oxidation occurs when there is oxygen present.

The following are the byproducts of each type of glucose oxidation:

- . Aerobic oxidation: Glucose completely oxidizes to produce 38 moles of energy, carbon dioxide, and water.

- Anaerobic oxidation: Lactic acid and carbon dioxide are produced as part of the partial oxidation of glucose to produce ethanol in plants and ethanol in animals. Two moles of energy are also produced.

3. Unexpected Blood Sugar Swings Reasons You Probably Didn't Know

Whether you have had type 2 diabetes for a short while or have had it for a longer period, you are aware of how unstable blood sugar levels may be and how crucial it is to maintain control over them.

To prevent potential diabetes complications like kidney disease, nerve damage, eye issues, stroke, and heart disease, proper blood sugar management is essential, according to the National Institutes of Health (NIH). Also, according to Lisa McDermott, RD, CDCES, a diabetes specialist with the Allegheny Health Network in Pittsburgh, maintaining your levels regularly helps keep you feeling energized, focused, and in a good mood.

According to the American Diabetes Association (ADA), taking the right medications, making smart food choices, exercising frequently, and having regular blood sugar checks can all help you maintain your levels within a healthy range. Before meals, the ADA advises keeping blood glucose levels between 80 and 130 milligrams per deciliter (mg/dL) and below 180 mg/dL two hours following the beginning of a meal. A1C tests, which assess your average blood glucose over the previous two to three months, are also advised by the organization to be taken at least twice annually if your blood sugar levels are stable and you are adhering to your treatment plan.

- **Dehydration Drives Up Blood Sugar**

Can a lack of fluids results in high blood sugar? True, and as it happens, the two are more closely related than you might think: According to McDermott, dehydration can cause hyperglycemia because it causes your blood sugar to become more concentrated. Even greater dehydration can arise from having high blood sugar, which can make you urinate more frequently.

To stay hydrated and healthy throughout the day, people with diabetes should be extremely watchful about drinking lots of water or other calorie-free beverages. The amount of water you should drink depends on your age and stage of life. Moreover, those with high levels of physical activity or body bulk have increased hydration requirements. If you have trouble drinking plain water, consider adding some citrus wedges, frozen berries, cucumber slices, or fresh mint leaves as a garnish. Unsweetened iced herbal teas, such as the raspberry, cherry, or peach flavors, are also incredibly cooling and devoid of caffeine, according to her.

• Artificial Sweeteners May Impact Blood Sugar Response

Because they believe that sugar-free drinks won't cause their blood sugar to rise, many diabetics seek diet drinks instead of ordinary soda or juice. However, a review that appeared in the January 2021 issue of Frontiers in Nutrition raised the possibility that artificial sweeteners could not be wholly neutral after all and might rather worsen glucose homeostasis.

Although most governmental and medical organizations say that most artificial sweeteners have no impact on blood sugar, the study is not conclusive in this regard. So what might be happening ? Those who consume artificial sugars may have a "rebound effect," according to the Mayo Clinic. They believe sugar-free food to be healthy, so they overindulge or consume other carb-heavy items because they believe the diet drink will allow them to "afford" it. The clinic also mentions the possibility of diarrhea from some noncaloric sweeteners, which can exacerbate dehydration.

Patty Bonsignore, RN, CDCES, a nurse educator at the Joslin Diabetes Center in Boston, advises those who frequently consume diet Coke to cut back and see if doing so affects their blood sugar levels. Use water or seltzer rather than ordinary soda or juice to keep things sugar-free.

- **Some Medications Meddle With Diabetes Control**

The prescription and over-the-counter medications you take to treat health problems besides diabetes can monkey with blood sugar levels. One example is steroids (used to treat inflammatory conditions, autoimmune disorders, and asthma), which can cause blood sugar to shoot up dramatically, McDermott says. Birth control pills, certain antidepressants and antipsychotics, some diuretics, and nasal decongestants may also cause higher-than-normal readings, while other drugs may lower blood sugar or make it more difficult to recognize signs of hypoglycemia, according to TriHealth. "Even cough drops can affect blood sugar levels," she says.

- **Beware the Notorious "Dawn Phenomenon"**

Even if your blood glucose level was in the normal range before you went to bed, it's not unusual to wake up with a high reading. According to the Mayo Clinic, between 2 and 8 a.m., you might be going through the "dawn phenomenon," which happens when the body prepares for waking up by generating cortisol and other chemicals.

These hormones reduce the body's sensitivity to insulin, which in diabetics might cause a blood sugar increase in the morning. Even if your reading was in the normal range when you went to bed, it's not unusual to wake up with a high blood sugar reading. According to the Mayo Clinic, you may be going through the "dawn phenomenon," which happens between 2 and 8 a.m. when the body prepares for waking up by releasing cortisol and other chemicals. These hormones reduce the body's sensitivity to insulin and, in those with diabetes, can cause a morning blood sugar increase.

- **Women's Menstrual Cycles Can Affect Blood Sugar**

According to Women's College Hospital, hormonal fluctuations during a woman's premenstrual phase might lead her blood sugars to become a little out of whack, as if cramping, bloating, and mood swings weren't terrible enough.

According to McDermott, while the effect differs from person to person, some diabetic women lose some of their sensitivity to insulin a week or two before their period, which can result in higher-than-normal blood sugar levels. Once or shortly after menstruation starts, readings usually return to normal. You could find it helpful to reduce the number of carbohydrates you eat during that time or fit in more exercise if you discover that your blood sugar levels are persistently high the week before your period, she advises. Just make sure to closely monitor your cycle and blood sugar levels to make sure this is the root of the problem. Discuss possible medication adjustments for hormonal changes with your doctor or diabetes educator if you take insulin.

• Lack of Sleep May Lead to Unbalanced Blood Sugar

Sleepless nights can negatively impact your blood sugar in addition to your mood and energy levels. According to a review written in December 2015 for the journal Diabetes Treatment, type 2 diabetics may experience difficulties with glucose regulation and insulin sensitivity if they don't get enough sleep.

Sleep is healing, says Bonsignore. Lack of sleep causes the body to experience chronic stress, and any time stress levels are up, blood sugar levels rise as well.

Regrettably, McDermott note that persons with type 2 diabetes frequently complain about having problems sleeping. The condition known as sleep apnea, in which breathing regularly starts and stops while you are asleep, is more common in people with high body mass indices.

Work to establish a regular sleep schedule where you go to bed and wake up at the same time each day to increase the quantity and quality of your sleep. Your objective should be to get seven to nine hours of sleep each night, as advised by the National Sleep Foundation. See a sleep medicine specialist for assistance if you still have difficulties falling asleep or think you may have sleep apnea (perhaps your partner has complained about your snoring?), advises Bonsignore.

- **Too much caffeine might cause a spike in blood sugar**

Up to 400 mg of caffeine per day is considered safe for most individuals, but those with diabetes may experience low or high blood sugar as a result of caffeine's potential to influence how insulin functions. According to earlier studies, excessive coffee use can raise blood sugar levels in people with diabetes. To further complicate matters, another study that was released in January 2015 in the Journal of Clinical and Diagnostic Research claimed that caffeine use could help the body manage blood sugar levels and lower the risk of complications from diabetes.

Depending on the individual, maybe. A single cup of coffee can cause blood sugar levels to surge in some type 2 diabetics while not affecting others, according to McDermott.

You can only watch how caffeine affects you by tracking your blood sugar levels. To evaluate if your glucose control improves, Bonsignore advises those who frequently experience blood sugar swings and who eat a lot of caffeinated beverages (which include diet soda in addition to coffee and tea).

• **Errors in Blood Sugar Testing May Lead to Unreliable Readings**

You risk getting a false alarm if you forget to wash your hands before monitoring your blood sugar. Research has revealed that testing after handling food can result in an incorrectly high value because sugar residues on the skin can contaminate the blood sample. You may wind up taking too much insulin if your blood sugar levels are higher than they are, Ms. Dermott warns. Dangerously low blood sugar levels were the outcome.

Due to the extremely small blood sample size used by modern blood sugar meters, it is possible to easily misjudge the glucose concentration in the sample. If you can't get to a faucet to wash your hands well, using the second drop of blood after wiping away the first will increase testing precision.

Chapter 2 : Why is glucose so important ?

Every cell in the human body needs the energy to carry out the metabolic processes necessary for life. Little, simple sugars like glucose are the main source of energy for the body's organs and tissues, including the brain, muscles, and many others. The body's major structural molecules, such as glycoproteins and glycolipids, are also constructed from glucose. The amount of glucose in the body is closely controlled. Serious, sometimes fatal problems emerge from abnormally high or low levels.

1. Mental Fuel

The majority of the brain's energy requirements are typically met by glucose. The brain requires a steady supply of glucose due to its high energy needs and inability to store the sugar. The body is made up of several

The metabolic processes that support life require energy, which is needed by every cell in the human body. A little, simple sugar called glucose is the main source of fuel for the body's energy production, particularly for the muscles, brain, and various other organs and tissues. Moreover, bigger structural molecules found in the body like glycoproteins and glycolipids are constructed from glucose. The glucose levels in the body are tightly controlled. Abnormally high or low levels cause severe, possibly fatal consequences.

2. Exercise Fuel

Depending on sex, age, and level of fitness, the skeletal muscles typically make up between 30 and 40 percent of the total body weight. During the activity, the skeletal muscles need a lot of glucose. Skeletal muscles store blood sugar in the form of glycogen, which is readily broken down to provide glucose during physical activity, in contrast to the brain. During activity, muscle tissue also often absorbs a significant amount of glucose from the bloodstream. Even though skeletal muscles can use molecules generated from fat as an energy source, the depletion of glucose reserves during prolonged activity can cause rapid exhaustion, also known as bonking or hitting the wall.

3. Other Tissues and Organs' Fuel

The body's numerous organs and tissues can use a variety of fuels. Some other significant organs and tissues, in addition to the brain and skeletal muscles, depend on glucose as their main or only fuel source. Examples include the red and white blood cells as well as the cornea, lens, and retina of the eyes. It's interesting to note that although the small intestine's cells are in charge of absorbing glucose from food and transferring it to the bloodstream, they mostly use glutamine as a fuel source. This frees up more glucose for other tissues and organs that depend on the sugar more.

4. Role structures

The human body uses glucose, along with other chemicals, to create other crucial structural components in addition to its function in energy production. One such instance is the glycoprotein collagen, which has a protein backbone as well as simple carbohydrates like glucose. Skin, muscles, bones, and other human tissues all contain collagen, an important structural component. The growth and upkeep of the body's nerves are significantly influenced by other glycoproteins. Glycolipids, which are made up of the building blocks of fat and sugar, are essential parts of the membranes that envelop and support each of the body's cells.

5. Diabetic Hyperglycemia and Hypoglycemia

Because of the brain's exquisite dependency on a steady supply of glucose, symptoms of hypoglycemia often appear rather rapidly after a considerable drop in blood sugar. Hyperglycemia, or a high blood sugar level, may or may not have overt symptoms. The combination of high blood sugar and lack of insulin frequently results in signs and symptoms such as extreme thirst and hunger accidental weight loss lack of energy increased urination in persons with type 1 diabetes, who produce little or no insulin.

These signs and symptoms frequently do not appear or are not noticeable in patients with type 2 diabetes or its precursor prediabetes. Due to this, many persons with these diseases can go years without receiving a diagnosis. Yet, despite the absence of symptoms, continuous hyperglycemia can result in serious side effects, including kidney and heart problems, nerve damage, and eye issues that could result in blindness.

6. Precautions and Warnings

Discuss any worries you may have about your blood glucose levels with your doctor because glucose performs so many crucial bodily tasks. This is crucial if you have any of the following risk factors for prediabetes and type 2 diabetes: age over 40 above-average body weight sedentary lifestyle parents or siblings who have the disease.

If you experience any hypoglycemic or hyperglycemic signs or symptoms, you should seek emergency medical assistance. If you have diabetes, be sure to closely adhere to your dietary, exercise, and medication programs. Unless your doctor instructs you to, don't stop taking your prescription or modify the dosage.

7. Sources

The body obtains the glucose it requires from food sources, bodily reserves of glycogen (the storage form of glucose), and gluconeogenesis, a process that creates glucose from other molecules. It's crucial to include healthy sources of glucose in a well-balanced diet because the body can only store enough glycogen to meet its energy requirements for about a half-day. overall objectives.

The following are typical target blood sugar ranges :

	Targets for blood sugar in those	Blood sugar levels that should be achieved by

	without diabetes	diabetics
Before meals	72–99 mg/dl	80–130 mg/dl
2 hours after a meal	less than 140 mg/dl	less than 180 mg/dl

Chapter 3 : How do plants manufacture glucose ?

1.   Photosynthesis example

Plants do not require the nourishment of other living or extinct species, as do animals. Instead, utilizing light energy, typically from the Sun, and straightforward inorganic elements, the majority of plants are able to produce their own sustenance in the form of a sugar called glucose. Carbon dioxide is needed for this activity, which is typically taken up by plants from the atmosphere through their leaves.

Furthermore, water molecules are needed for this activity, which are typically taken up from the soil by a plant's roots. The majority of a plant's glucose is created in the leaves, which is where this water is often transferred up the stem of the plant.

Carbon dioxide and water combine when exposed to light energy to create glucose, which may be used by cells to produce energy. As well as oxygen, which is either released back into the atmosphere or consumed in respiration. Photosynthesis is the process by which glucose is produced in the presence of light energy and basic inorganic molecules.

The prefix photo- denotes the need for light energy in this reaction, while the suffix -synthesis denotes the creation or synthesis of something through this reaction. We now know that glucose is the chemical that is being created.

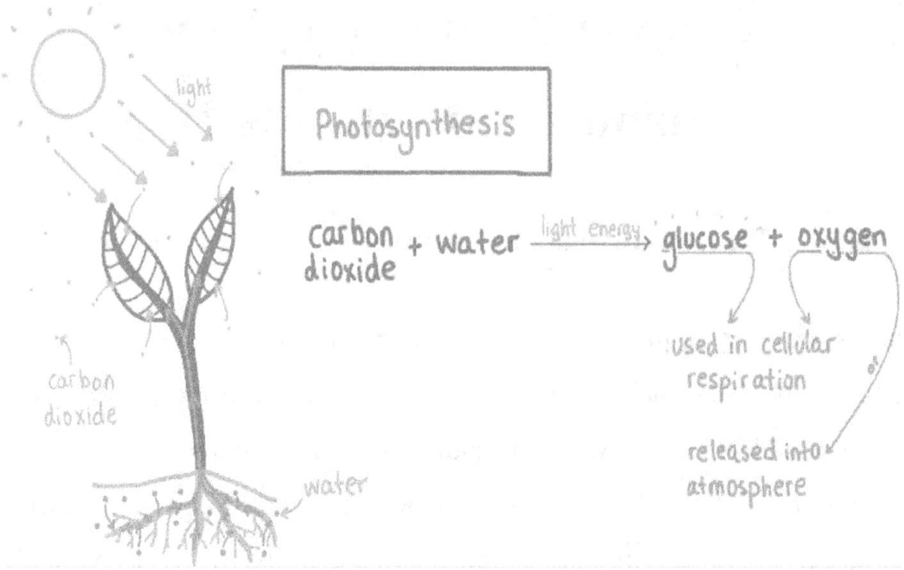

2. Overall photosynthesis response

Photosynthesis is an oxidation-reduction reaction that is light-enhanced. (Reduction refers to a molecule gaining electrons; oxidation refers to the removal of electrons from a molecule.) As a plant engages in photosynthesis, light energy is used to propel the oxidation of water (H2O), resulting in the production of oxygen gas (O2), hydrogen ions (H+), and electrons. The majority of the hydrogen ions and removed electrons finally migrate to carbon dioxide (CO2), which is then reduced to organic compounds.

In addition to hydrogen ions, extra electrons are required for the reduction of nitrate and sulfate to amino and sulfhydryl groups in amino acids, the building blocks of proteins. The primary direct organic products of photosynthesis in the majority of green cells are starch and sucrose. The typical reaction in which (CH2O) type carbohydrates are produced during photosynthesis in plants can be represented by the equation below:

3.   The effectiveness of photosynthesis in terms of energy

The ratio of energy stored to energy from light absorbed is the energy efficiency of photosynthesis. The difference between the energy contained in gaseous oxygen and organic materials is the chemical energy stored. The ratio of energy stored to energy from light absorbed is the energy efficiency of photosynthesis. The chemical energy stored is different from the energy present in water, carbon dioxide, and other reactants, as well as the energy present in gaseous oxygen and organic compound products. The number of products generated, which varies depending on the plant species and environmental factors, makes it impossible to know exactly how much energy is stored. The synthesis of one mole (i.e., 6.02 1023 molecules; abbreviated N) of oxygen and one-sixth mole of glucose results in the storage of approximately 117 kilocalories (kcal) of chemical energy, according to the equation for glucose formation provided earlier. The efficiency of photosynthesis can then be determined by comparing this amount to the amount of light required to produce one mole of oxygen.

Chapter 4 : A Blood Glucose Level: What Is It?

1. Blood Glucose Fonction

The blood contains a form of sugar called glucose, which gives your body's cells energy. As you eat, your blood glucose levels rise and then fall as your body produces insulin to assist in transferring the sugar from your bloodstream to your cells. To prevent blood sugar from dips if too much time elapses between meals, the liver intervenes and releases glucose that has been stored. The overarching objective is to consistently maintain your blood glucose level within the normal range.

Your blood glucose level is one of the most crucial measurements in your body when it comes to sustaining your health. Blood glucose, also referred to as blood sugar, gives your body the energy it needs to power the brain, heart, and muscles. The majority of the glucose in your body is derived from meals, but some are also made by the liver and utilized as needed. Ideally, your blood glucose level ranges from 80 to 99 mg/dL (milligrams of sugar per deciliter of blood) during the day, with transitory rises after meals followed by insulin-aided reductions back into the normal range.

2. Normal Levels of Blood Glucose

Your age, life expectancy, and medical history are a few of the elements that affect what your optimal blood glucose level should be. Your typical fasting blood sugar level, if you do not have diabetes of any kind, should be between 80 and 99 mg/dL, with a potential rise to 140 mg/dL immediately after eating. With a potential jump to 180 mg/dL after eating, your tolerable fasting blood sugar level may be greater if you have been diagnosed with diabetes, at 80 to 130 mg/dL.

3. Sugar Levels with Diabetes

The pancreas sometimes struggles to complete its job properly. Diabetes patients either generate very little or no insulin, or they produce it in extremely small amounts and are resistant to its effects. Diabetes develops when glucose from the meals we eat merely builds up in the bloodstream rather than converting to energy as it should. This can happen if insulin isn't released into the bloodstream or doesn't function properly.

The most severe cases of diabetes require insulin replacement therapy to maintain blood glucose levels under control. Although drugs and insulin may be required for good control, diet modifications, and exercise can help manage diabetes in less severe instances.

You will need to monitor your blood glucose levels multiple times a day, typically before and after meals, if you develop diabetes. This aids in figuring out how many carbohydrates you can eat at each meal as well as how much insulin or medication you should take. Using a glucose meter at home is the most typical technique to check your blood sugar level. You can use these tools to apply a little drop of blood to a test strip that slides into the meter. After analyzing the blood sample, it displays the blood glucose level.

4.   High blood sugar symptoms and complications

The medical word for a transiently elevated blood glucose level in a diabetic patient is hyperglycemia. This may occur if you overeat, forget to take your insulin or oral diabetic medicine, or get sick. If you have diabetes, especially Type 1 diabetes, a high blood sugar level can have detrimental effects. If your blood sugar isn't brought down, it can cause diabetic ketoacidosis, a potentially fatal illness that might put you in a coma. Frequent urination, excessive thirst, recurrent infections, hazy vision, irritability, and weariness are all signs of high blood sugar.

5.   Low blood sugar symptoms and complications

The signs of hypoglycemia, which occur when your blood glucose level goes too low, frequently include headache, trembling, sweating, clamminess, increased appetite, irritability, and confusion. These signs and symptoms might emerge unexpectedly and are typically the result of skipping meals. Seizures and even unexpected death are possible outcomes. You can quickly elevate your blood sugar level by consuming fast-acting carbs like fruit juice, honey, glucose pills, and hard candies.

6. Who Is Responsible for Blood Glucose Levels ?

Anybody who exhibits high blood sugar or low blood sugar symptoms should see a doctor to have their blood glucose level evaluated. Anybody with known endocrine disorders, such as hypoglycemia and diabetes, must undoubtedly keep an eye on their blood sugar levels as part of their medical care. Pregnant women and those who have major risk factors, such as a long family history of diabetes or obesity mixed with a sedentary lifestyle, should also monitor their blood sugar levels.

7.   Which Individuals Should Monitor Blood Glucose Levels ?

Anyone who exhibits signs of high or low blood sugar should see a doctor to have their blood glucose level evaluated. To treat their ailment, people with recognized endocrine diseases like diabetes and hypoglycemia must keep an eye on their blood sugar levels. Pregnant women and individuals with major risk factors, such as a long family history of diabetes or obesity mixed with a sedentary lifestyle, are two more distinct groups of people who should monitor their blood sugar levels.

Chapter 5 : Blood Sugar Control, Menopause, and Weight Management

1. Resistant to Insulin

The amount of glucose (blood sugar) in a person's body can be managed with the aid of the hormone insulin. The primary fuel used by the body is glucose. Once glucose enters the body's cells, insulin draws it from the bloodstream. When the cells in the muscles, body fat, and liver ignore or reject insulin's signaling efforts, insulin resistance develops.

High blood sugar, or an excessive amount of glucose circulating through the bloodstream, results from the body's cells not appropriately responding to insulin signals. Weight Increase Associated with Menopause and Estrogen. Weight gain is a common side effect of menopause for women. While estrogen helps insulin function optimally, this is often caused by a deficiency. Throughout each step of the menopause process, a woman's production of estrogen and progesterone gradually decreases over time. The risk of the body developing insulin resistance increases as a result.

As estrogen levels fall, a woman's appetite frequently increases because estrogen also affects the signals that indicate hunger and satiety. A menopausal woman who previously had no real problems with overeating or identifying when she was truly hungry may discover that she is continuously hungry and consumes a lot more calories, which leads to weight gain. A woman may notice changes in how her body distributes fat when the levels of estrogen and progesterone decline throughout menopause. Weight gain may start to build up in the abdominal area, leading to a larger belly, rather than around a woman's hips or thighs. Visceral fat is the type of fat that is frequently referred to as "menopause belly." Retinol-binding protein 4 is a protein that is secreted by visceral fat and is linked to insulin resistance. Moreover, Type 2 diabetes can develop as a result of high visceral fat levels.

2. Factors that Increase Menopausal Weight

Many risk factors have been linked to menopausal weight gain. Some of these elements are physiological and are regarded as immutable. Yet, there are numerous ways to change other risk factors that are psychological and lifestyle-related.

3. Physiological Considerations

• Aging

• Decline in lean mass and basal metabolic rate (BMR): It is frequently noted that excessive weight gain over a short period coincides with a reduction in lean mass. A menopausal woman may find it difficult to burn calories efficiently enough to keep a proper caloric balance as her metabolic rate slows down.

• Secondary causes : Musculoskeletal problems like osteoporosis or osteoarthritis, hypothyroidism, or conditions like polycystic ovarian syndrome (PCOS) can all be identified as a primary contributing factor to menopausal weight increase.

4. Psychological Considerations

• Negative emotional state (depression, stress, worry, mood disorders): Menopausal women may encounter several types of psychological suffering, which are frequently impacted or sparked by concerns about one's appearance. There are numerous physical changes associated with menopause over time, and some women may find these changes to be particularly emotionally taxing.

• Emotional eating: As food provides comfort, some menopausal women may use food to cope with their uncertainties and difficulties.

5. Variables related to lifestyle

It includes High-calorie intake, excessive sugar and processed food intake, inactivity, sleep deprivation, use of tobacco and alcohol, and low dietary fiber. For menopausal women, these lifestyle elements combine to produce a "perfect storm" of worries. Consuming good food is equally as important as eating a lot of it. The quality of the food is equally important, even though calorie intake is a major factor in hormonal weight growth. The body will not be properly nourished if you eat a diet high in processed foods, sugar, bad fats, and salt, which will result in weight gain. Lack of sufficient nutrition might make you lethargic and provide you with little energy for daily activities like exercise. Sleep patterns may also be disturbed as a result of this. During and After Menopause Blood Sugar Management Recommendations

The key to preventing weight gain during menopause and beyond is proper blood sugar stabilization and continued blood glucose management.

6. Low-Carbohydrate Diet

For women in menopause and postmenopause, a low-carb diet that reduces glucose intake is strongly advised. Consuming fewer carbohydrates can significantly improve blood sugar control and weight loss. A nutrient-rich diet rich in wholesome foods like grass-fed meat, fish, fruits, vegetables, raw dairy, fermented foods, seeds, and healthy fats will not only help you feel full and content but will also help you avoid cravings and maintain stable blood sugar levels.

In addition to eating a diet high in nutrients, it's crucial to stay away from processed foods that are high in sugar, inflammatory industrial seed oils, and artificial additives. These dietary items not only trigger cravings and leave the body unsatisfied, but they also raise blood sugar levels and put the body under stress.

It is crucial to understand that a diet high in nutrients and free of processed foods does not necessarily equate to one that is low in calories. Calorie restriction has been associated with a decrease in metabolic rate, which can lead to weight gain and insulin resistance. Food that is properly prepared is fuel.

7. Exercise

Maintaining steady glucose levels requires regular exercise. The body may benefit from guidance on how to use insulin effectively. During menopause, women may become less active for a variety of reasons, including physical restrictions, fatigue, and lifestyle changes that no longer call for them to be as active daily. Making time throughout your day to move your body can be quite beneficial.

Depending on one's physical capabilities and preferred methods, regular exercise can be done in a variety of ways to help the body burn sugar. Blood sugar levels can be kept consistent throughout the day with just a small amount of exercise, such as walking for 30 minutes a day or 10 to 20 minutes after each meal. The addition of resistance training exercises can assist preserve bone density and mass and prevent problems like osteoporosis. Additional moderate aerobic exercises like swimming, jogging, or bicycling can help offer diversity to an exercise regimen. Daily exercise can also aid in balancing calorie intake and easing common menopausal symptoms like hot flashes and trouble sleeping.

8.   Establish Appropriate Thyroid Function

The thyroid hormone is influenced by estrogen levels after menopause in a cellular manner, which might affect metabolic health. The thyroid gland produces insufficient thyroid hormone, which causes hypothyroidism. Menopausal women may experience additional weight issues as a result of the metabolism slowing down as a result of this. A qualified healthcare professional should do a complete thyroid panel and be able to address any imbalances.

9. Berberine and cinnamon dietary supplement

Blood sugar regulation can be greatly aided by taking supplements of cinnamon and berberine. Plants like Phellodendron, European barberry, and goldenseal contain the chemical berberine, which has historically been utilized in Chinese and Ayurveda medicine. Berberine assists the body in developing efficient insulin processing, which awakens fat-burning enzymes and gradually reduces body fat by activating the AMPK protein.

Blood sugar levels can be effectively managed by using cinnamon. By including a tiny bit of this common aromatic spice in liquids, smoothies, or other dishes daily, one can easily include it in their diet. Cinnamon increases insulin sensitivity and slows the breakdown of carbohydrates, preventing a blood sugar surge in the body. It is advised to only eat up to a teaspoon of Ceylon cinnamon or about a quarter of a teaspoon of cassia every day.

10.   Hydration

Daily hydration aids in flushing extra blood sugar out of the body through the urine and kidneys. It is advised to drink water that has been thoroughly filtered, and it is advantageous to add a pinch of unrefined salt to assist maintain the right balance of minerals and electrolytes.

11.   Stress Management

The best way to maintain healthy blood sugar levels is to handle stress daily. The body produces more glucose as cortisol levels start to rise in response to stress.

It is crucial to work to identify the sources of stress and, whenever practical, try to reduce or eliminate those stresses. Even while it might not always be an option, there are many other ways to deal with stress, such as going outside and doing your favorite activity, talking to a loved one or therapist about your stress, and making time each day for prayer or meditation. To handle daily stress and reduce anxiety, finding strategies for deep relaxation, such as breathing exercises or yoga, can be beneficial.

A woman's blood sugar levels should be closely monitored during her menopausal years to detect any insulin resistance concerns and determine what might be causing glucose spikes.

Chapter 6 : Dietary recommendations to prevent, manage, and reverse type 2 diabetes

1. Dietary recommendations for type 2 diabetes prevention, management, and reversal

Choosing what to eat after receiving a type 2 diabetes diagnosis may be one of the most difficult issues. It is crucial to actively participate in the creation of your treatment plan, actively seek information, and actively educate yourself in this area because diet plays such a significant role.

2. Consume food that is low in saturated fats.

When fat from the circulation accumulates inside muscle cells, it produces harmful breakdown products (free radicals) that lead to inflammation and mitochondrial dysfunction. This occurrence is known as lipotoxicity. All of these procedures stop the "insulin-signaling" function, which causes blood sugar levels to rise.

By injecting fat into people's blood and seeing how their "insulin resistance" increased noticeably, researchers were able to demonstrate how fat affects how "insulin function" works. On the other hand, "insulin resistance" declines when fat is removed from the bloodstream. MRI technology may often be used to track the association between fat transferring from the bloodstream to the muscles and the corresponding level of "insulin resistance"

Type 2 diabetes is directly affected by the fats palmitate (palmitic acid) and oleate (oleic acid) :

• Palmitic acid, a saturated fat that is included in meat, dairy products, and eggs and which reduces insulin release, raises insulin resistance and may be harmful to pancreatic cells.

• Oleic acid, a monosaturated lipid that can be found in nuts, olives, and avocados, may help to prevent diabetes.

The Epic-Panacea study, one of the largest investigations on the relationship between meat consumption and body weight, demonstrates that, on average, if two people consume the same number of calories, the person eating more meat acquires noticeably more weight.

The same study concluded that poultry may be the meat that causes people to gain the most weight, finding that over fourteen years, people's BMI (Body Mass Index) grew in proportion to the amount of fowl they consumed.

3.　Eat legumes since they can aid with blood sugar regulation

Individuals that consume a lot of legumes (beans, chickpeas, and lentils) are typically lighter in weight. This diet has been found to have the same results as calorie restriction in terms of weight loss and blood sugar regulation, with the added advantages of better cholesterol and "insulin regulation". Several studies have demonstrated the positive effects of fenugreek, fava beans (Vicia faba), and mung beans on lowering blood sugar and cholesterol levels.

4.   Plants that improve the control of diabetes

Blood sugar levels are lowered by the "wonder plant" moringa oleifera. Three human studies and two animal research have demonstrated the beneficial effects of Moringa oliefera leaves on type 2 diabetes by lowering cholesterol, reducing inflammation, and safeguarding pancreatic cells. Moringa also contains four of the phytochemicals with the greatest influence on hyperglycemia and dyslipidemia.

When compared to the research groups that did not get any Moringa oleifera supplementation, the groups who received a daily dose of Moringa oleifera leaf powder showed considerably lower levels of diabetes indicators. Also, it has been demonstrated that a mixture of phytochemicals from cranberry, oregano, rosemary, and Rhodiola rosea is effective in the treatment of diabetes and the enhancement of pancreatic function.

Also, research on people has indicated that eating algae can lower the chance of developing diabetes, while research on animals has revealed that Chlorella vulgaris may prevent the emergence of "insulin resistance" and that marine spirulina drastically changes the symptoms of diabetes. It has been demonstrated that a diet rich in zinc and spirulina has positive effects on cholesterol, blood sugar, and triglyceride levels.

Cinnamon may be a good alternative for controlling blood glucose and blood pressure, according to randomized, placebo-controlled, and double-blind human trials.

In one study, for instance, consuming at least 2 grams of cinnamon daily for 12 weeks dramatically decreased the primary diabetes indicators.

5.   Avoid processed cereals, sweetened beverages, and treats

Beyond abstaining from meat and saturated fats, there are other suggestions for preventing and treating type 2 diabetes. A 2016 study that evaluated the connection between dietary practices and health status in over 200 000 persons found that people who consume an unhealthy plant-based diet are more likely to develop type 2 diabetes.

Conclusion

Diabetes develops when blood sugar levels remain elevated, which may damage blood vessels. The vital organs that are supplied by these vessels as a result are also impacted. Diabetes can cause renal failure, amputation of the lower extremities, eyesight loss, circulation issue, and even death. It has been established that intensive pharmacological therapy is unsuccessful in treating the condition and can even be fatal in some cases. Yet studies have revealed that a plant-based diet and considerable lifestyle adjustments can help control and even reverse chronic illness. The focus should be placed on balancing the levels of "insulin" in patients with type 2 diabetes (the hormone that helps the cells in the body take up glucose from the blood). If too much fat is accumulated in muscle cells as a result of refined carbohydrates, organic pollutants, inflammatory conditions inside the body, and a lack of exercise, the hormone's ability to function is reduced. A vegan or vegetarian diet decreases blood sugar levels, aids in achieving and maintaining a healthy BMI (Body Mass Index), and lessens the effects of organic pollutants and inflammation on our bodies. It also helps the "insulin-hormone" operate again.